Coming Back Home, A Dementia Experience

Introduction

My wife, Kathy, had early-onset dementia at the age of 62. This book is an account of our 10 year experience with dementia that was diagnosed to be Frontal-Temporal (FTD). Kathy had the additional problem of being gluten and dairy intolerant. Documented are our experiences with prescription drugs, Memory Care Facilities, and the use of natural supplements in place of prescription drugs in order to bring Kathy back home. Kathy has now been off of prescription drugs and back home for 18 months.

The Beginning

Kathy's early-onset dementia story begins about 10 years ago at age 62. At the time, her blood pressure was on the high side, typically 145/70. However, whenever we would go in to see the doctor, it would be 160-170/70 (white coat syndrome). Kathy was very afraid and had a lot of anxiety about having a stroke because of the perceived high blood pressure. In any event, she ended up being given two prescription drugs: Lisinopril (20mg x2) to reduce blood pressure, and and a diuretic, hydrochorothiazide (12.5mg). Kathy first tried a beta-blocker for BP, but her pulse dropped too low and I was afraid that she might pass out. We had always been anti-drugs, so this was hard to accept. However, at this point, I didn't know of a quick solution using natural alternatives. Things to try longer term, but no quick fix.

Actually, her story begins about 20 years earlier when we determined that she was gluten and dairy intolerant, but not celiac. The gluten intolerance would result in migraine-like headaches. This was assumed to be an autoimmune response that caused brain inflammation. Because of lactose intolerance, dairy had already being minimized because it caused upset stomach and severe constipation. However, we weren't strict until Kathy began having neurological problems, then we started a strict no-gluten and no-dairy diet.

One explanation for the headaches is that the gluten peptide and the dairy casein peptides look similar to some of the brain cells and therefore the immune system was also attacking the brain cells thus causing the inflammation.

Although Kathy had been taking the two prescription drugs for several months, they seemed to have little effect on her blood pressure (BP) that we were monitoring at home. Her anxiety grew worse and she began to have the white coat syndrome even at home.

As a result, it was a fateful weekend when we went to the Urgent Care Center to get something for her anxiety. That something was a prescription drug Clonazepam (0.5mg), a benzodiazepine that acts on GABA receptors. Thus, much to my dismay, Kathy was now taking three prescription drugs.

As mentioned, Kathy's neurological problems started about 10 years ago This is also the about the same time that she began taking the prescription drugs.

The Symptoms Start

The first neurological symptom was when she had trouble following text when reading and Kathy started trying to use her figure as a guide.

Then she started having trouble writing.

Then she had trouble with speech and locating objects close to her.

At the time, we were living on a small lake in a rural area. The nearest hospital was a half hour away and the nearest family doctor was about 15 minutes away. It was obvious that this location would not be adequate for her worsening condition and therefore we moved to a large city where specialists were available and family nearby. However, before we left, an MRI was done at the regional hospital. The MRI machines are very noisy and luckily we were able to get Kathy to remain still.

The MRI showed that there was significant damage to the parietal portion of the brain as well as some of the frontal lobe. Internet source www.neuroskills.com claims that:

*"If **damage** is sustained to the **parietal lobe**, a person would most likely have difficulty reading, recognizing people and objects, and having a comprehensive awareness of his or her own body and limbs and their positioning in space."*
and,

*"**Damage** to the left **parietal lobe** can result in what is called "Gerstmann's Syndrome." It includes right-left confusion, difficulty with writing (agraphia) and difficulty with mathematics*

(acalculia). It can also produce disorders of language (aphasia) and the inability to perceive objects normally (agnosia)."

Although her ocular vision was fine, she began having trouble locating objects near her and as a result she began having trouble holding a fork and eating normally. The neuron signals from the eyes were no longer being processed correctly by the brain.

As her memory faded, taking the medications became a problem. I did not know whether she was taking 1, 2, or no pills. I had to start taking control of her dosage. And, since I felt that the medications were somehow related to her neurological problems, I wanted to start weaning her off of them.

Since the BP drugs seemed to have little effect on her BP, I started there. The easiest one to discontinue was the diuretic since it was not taken every day. The Lisinopril was quite another matter. Kathy was absolutely insistent on taking it. As a solution, I went to the drug store to find a pill that looked like the Lisinopril. It turned out that baby aspirin looked similar and I substituted those in the prescription bottle. I was no longer concerned about her taking the substituted BP medication. At her insistence, I would periodically check her BP and, even if a little high, I would always tell her that it was good. It had been a couple years, but I had finally gotten her off the BP medicine.

Backing Up for a Minute

I believe Kathy had double jeopardy. It is conceivable that she had two separate, but possibly related paths to dementia:

1. Gluten and dairy intolerance
2. Prescription drugs to treat anxiety and high blood pressure.

As mentioned earlier, gluten, and dairy to a lesser extent, caused migraine-like headaches. The gluten peptides and the dairy casein peptides look very similar to some of the brain cells and therefore the immune system was attacking the brain cells thus causing the inflammation. It is my belief that this inflammation would lead to late-onset dementia, whereas the medications caused early-onset dementia. Kathy's mother died of late-onset dementia, which may have been caused by an intolerance to gluten and/or dairy.

Over the past 5 years or so, if she eats gluten and dairy, she becomes very agitated and uncontrollable. This is evidence of a gluten-neurological connection.

Continuing to Decline

Kathy's memory and mood continued to decline. She started waking up violently and throwing off the covers in a panic. She was afraid of the green light on the ceiling smoke detector. I covered that with tape. Fortunately, she got over being afraid of the ceiling fan.

Then urinating and bowel movements not in the bathroom began. Finally Kathy had to start wearing incontinence underwear.

Kathy would then have periods of extreme agitation, paranoia, and was at times uncontrollable. I had to learn the hard way that wine and alcohol significantly interfere with the Clonazepam effectiveness.

Kathy began to wander and several times our family had to drive out and search for her. The local police department became very familiar with Kathy also. The police picked her up walking beside the road in the rain about a half mile away. There were a couple more instances. I had bought her a bracelet with her information on it in cause she became lost. Another time, she road her bicycle down to the southern edge of our town. Fortunately, I received a call when the people noticed a problem.

And one night, she got out and was knocking on neighbor's doors at 4:00 in the morning. Fortunately, no one responded before I caught up with her.

Her periods of memory loss, agitation, and paranoia continued to grow worse. It became aggravating beyond belief to be constantly searching for her purse. She would hide it at home because of her paranoia, and forget it at restaurants. I finally reduced her credit card to a very low limit and made a copy of her license to put it in the purse.

Understanding Clonazapam's uses can help in understanding Kathy's behavior. Clonazapam is used to control:

1. Anxiety
2. Short term memory loss after surgery

3. Seizures

This medication was intended only for short term use (2 weeks) and not intended for long term use. Thus, although Kathy was being treated for anxiety, memory loss was a side effect. And, unfortunately, as indicated by the quote from the Clonazapam Addiction Help Website:

"Is Memory Loss Permanent?
While memory loss is a common side effect of clonazepam use, the symptoms are likely to cease when a person ends their short-term use. However, prolonged and excessive use of the drug can cause brain damage that might be irreversible. It is important to get treatment for clonazepam abuse to prevent any brain damage, physical damage, or further psychological harm."

Sadly, it is my position that the the result of long term Clonazapam use by Kathy did result in her early-onset dementia. I sometimes blame myself for not getting her off of this drug quicker. However, anxiety was still a problem and she was already addicted to it at this point. Trying to reduce the dosage would make her behavior worse. Thus, I was always confronted with the question "was her condition actually that worsened state and the medication was helping, or was her behavior a result of the medication?" I asked the family doctor about getting her off of the medication, but he said because the dosage was so low and seemed to be helping her, then why not continue?

It came to the point where Kathy could no longer drive. The last time that she drove, she turned left in front of an oncoming car, which sent her to the hospital and totaled the car. Fortunately, Kathy had no serious injuries. This was the last time that she drove. Kathy was too afraid to drive after that.

One of the purposes of Clonazepam is to induce short-term memory loss. It was not clear whether she should take the pill in the morning, mid-day, or evening. Over a period of time, we settled on evening.

This is when the major issue arose. At times, Kathy would not know who I was and she thought I was someone off the street wanting to take her food, money, etc. I had to physically prevent her from leaving the house at 4:00 am once because she was going to go knock on neighbor's doors. She was afraid of me.

Reading more about the side effects of Clonazapam on the internet, I realized the Clonazapam was causing her not to know me. And since I was giving it to her in the evening, nighttime was the worst situation. I tried to wean her off of the Clonazepam by taking a file and reducing the tablet size little by little each week. Remember, this drug is more addictive than heroin, and more difficult to get off of.

The pill shaving lead to a near disaster. One morning Kathy had an absolute meltdown and was uncontrollable. To this day, I'm not sure how I was able to get her to take another pill. She finally calmed down a little later. To stop taking Clonazapam could cause a seizure or even death because the natural GABA had been displaced and there was not enough natural GABA receptors remaining to control the Glutamate.

Kathy was also prescribed Aricept (5mg) by the neurologist. This was taken for only a short time since I saw no difference in her condition, and it does not aide in recovery.

During all this experience, I still questioned whether her behavior was a result of the medication, or was it simply her underlying condition and the Clonazapam was helping to control it?

First Memory Care Facility

It was at this point that I decided that I could no longer take care of Kathy and I decided to move her to a Memory Care Facility (MCF). I did this for her own safety. This was about 4 years ago.

The first MCF that Kathy was moved into was located nearby. The Facility was new but the Memory Care unit was rather small. Kathy is very active and size became an issue. Leaving my soul mate of 46 years there was a very, very traumatic experience. I cried as I drove out of the parking lot. That emotion was so strong, that even to this day, I cry a little bit when I think of it.

One day when I came back in, she was sitting and crying looking out the window. That made my heart sink. Apparently, she had tried to get out of one of the locked doors and they wouldn't let her as expected. The fact that there was no one trying to console her really upset me. I took her back home that day. The size of the facility was also a factor in that decision.

Reading more about the side effects of Clonazapam on the internet, I realized the Clonazapam was causing her not to know me. And since I was giving it to her in the evening, nighttime was the worst situation. I tried to wean her off of the Clonazepam by taking a file and reducing the tablet size little by little each week. Remember, this drug is more addictive than heroin, and more difficult to get off of.

The pill shaving lead to a near disaster. One morning Kathy had an absolute meltdown and was uncontrollable. To this day, I'm not sure how I was able to get her to take another pill. She finally calmed down a little later. To stop taking Clonazapam could cause a seizure or even death because the natural GABA had been displaced and there was not enough natural GABA receptors remaining to control the Glutamate.

Kathy was also prescribed Aricept (5mg) by the neurologist. This was taken for only a short time since I saw no difference in her condition, and it does not aide in recovery.

During all this experience, I still questioned whether her behavior was a result of the medication, or was it simply her underlying condition and the Clonazapam was helping to control it?

First Memory Care Facility

It was at this point that I decided that I could no longer take care of Kathy and I decided to move her to a Memory Care Facility (MCF). I did this for her own safety. This was about 4 years ago.

The first MCF that Kathy was moved into was located nearby. The Facility was new but the Memory Care unit was rather small. Kathy is very active and size became an issue. Leaving my soul mate of 46 years there was a very, very traumatic experience. I cried as I drove out of the parking lot. That emotion was so strong, that even to this day, I cry a little bit when I think of it.

One day when I came back in, she was sitting and crying looking out the window. That made my heart sink. Apparently, she had tried to get out of one of the locked doors and they wouldn't let her as expected. The fact that there was no one trying to console her really upset me. I took her back home that day. The size of the facility was also a factor in that decision.

Our family located a larger, better equipped MCF that would be more suitable for Kathy.

Second Memory Care Facility

One of the goals when Kathy entered the new MCF was to have the the doctor do a systematic withdrawal from Clonazapam, which was something I tried but as previously mentioned nearly ended in disaster. Upon entering the MCF, she was mistakenly prescribed 0.5mg twice a day by the family doctor. It took me a little while to get that straightened out, but it was not a good start. She was transitioned initially to Effexor. However, other medications soon were added to try to control Kathy's behavior. Whether these were better or worse is debatable.

While at the MCF, Kathy had a variety of issues which included insomnia, incidents of aggression, agitation, and wandering. A major issue was that Kathy would sometimes go a couple days without sleeping. The neurologist would periodically experiment with different medication combinations to try and find the best combination for the current situation. During her stay, Kathy knocked one of the aides on her butt, and another aide was off of work for a week with a twisted shoulder. They soon found out that Kathy, although small, was quite strong and had upper body strength from swimming all her life.

The doctor at the MCF would routinely schedule urinary tract infection tests because of Kathy's insomnia. The results were always negative and when he then wanted to do a catheter, I said no, and that I would not approve any more urinary tests.

Kathy loved music and she used to play the piano. Although she no longer could read music, she still played beautiful chords and would sing in her own way. I would use my iPad and bluetooth speaker to play the old songs that she loved and sometimes for the other residents as well.

I was constantly washing soiled bedsheets, bedspreads and clothes. Cleaning the rug at the MCF was a common occurrence. The apartment was flooded several times. This is a consequence of having 15 or more residents to 1 aide at night.

I often took Kathy out to the park for a walk during the day and sometimes packed a lunch or ate out. This became increasing more difficult and a couple times she resisted going back into the facility and I had to call for help. The head nurse requested that I not take her out for awhile.

After a period of time in the MCF, Kathy was taking the following cocktail of prescription drugs (descriptions from www.Drugs.com):

1. *Pyridostigmine BR 60mg Tablet (Mestinon)*

"An orally active cholinesterase inhibitor. Pyridostigmine bromide inhibits the destruction of acetylcholine by cholinesterase and thereby permits freer transmission of nerve impulses across the neuromuscular junction."

2. *Divalproex SOD 125mg Cap (DB)*

"Divalproex sodium affects chemicals in the body that may be involved in causing seizures. It is also used to treat manic episodes related to bipolar disorder (manic depression), and to prevent migraine headaches. Unfortunately, the anticonvulsant medication has been linked to suicide, liver toxicity, and pancreatitis. Divalproex works by increasing the amount of the neurotransmitter gamma amminobutyric acid (GABA) in the brain."

3. Venlafaxine HCL 37.5 mg Tablet (Effexor)

"Venlafaxine is an antidepressant in a group of drugs called selective serotonin and norepinephrine reuptake inhibitors (SSNRIs). Venlafaxine affects chemicals in the brain that may be unbalanced in people with depression. It is used to treat major depressive disorder, anxiety, and panic disorder."

4. Amantadine 50mg/5 ml Syrup

"Amantadine prevents and treats certain types of flu. It is used to treat Parkinson disease and uncontrolled muscle movements caused by some medicines. How amantadine works against Parkinson disease is not known."

As we know, prescription drugs do have side effects. The literature suggests the average number of side effects for drugs is approximately 70, whereas for for brain medications it is over 200. Although prescription drugs may work as intended most of the time, at times they created the very problem that was being treated. Kathy had instances of aggression and that would be treated with even more medications. My experience has been that it always results in a downward spiral of more and more medications.

The last medication to be added to her prescriptions was Amantadine. This was my least favorite. The Amantadine made Kathy drowsy and almost unresponsive to me. It was questionable whether it was worth my time to go see her because it made no difference. Also, when she would sleep, she would jerk and shake, which certainly wasn't quality sleep. I asked the nurse to please have the doctor reduce the dosage, which they did. I was a frequent visitor to the head nurse's office trying to get the medications reduced to minimize the negative effects on Kathy. However, I understood their position of needing to insure that residents and staff members were safe, and that she would not be disruptive.

Increasing medications did result in large purple patches under the skin of the forearms and hands which were of concern. Hallucinations were ever present.

I received a call one day that Kathy had slapped another resident. I was told that the Neurologist at the MCF had no further medications to recommend and that she would have to leave or go to a Psychiatric Hospital to to have her medications adjusted. If the medication change was successful, she could then return after having been a resident for almost 2 years. I didn't have much choice but to agree.

Psychiatric Hospital

This Hospital is where they typically treat people with alcohol and drug addiction, suicidal tendencies, manic depression, schizophrenia, etc. What a disaster! The handoff of medications between the MCF and the Clinic did not occur. As a result, Kathy suffered withdrawal while at the Clinic and they gave her PRN shots that turned out to be a benzodiazapine. Although she was being watched 24 hours, and trying to sleep in a bed intended for suicidal patients, she still fell down and hit her head. As a precaution, she was sent to the hospital for a CAT scan where they had to give her another PRN shot to calm her down. The scan was negative.

The medication chosen for Kathy by the Hospital medical staff was Zyprexa. I do not know what the dosage was. A description of this medication is as follows:

"Zyprexa (olanzapine) is an antipsychotic medication that affects chemicals in the brain. Zyprexa is used to treat the symptoms of psychotic conditions such as schizophrenia and bipolar disorder. Zyprexa is a *thienobenzodiazepine. This drug blocks multiple receptors, including dopamine and serotonin in the brain. It is not approved by the FDA (Off-Label) for use in psychotic conditions related to dementia. It may increase the risk of death in older adults with dementia-related conditions."*

Sounds like a good choice, don't you think?

Our initial shock was when our family first went to to see her during visiting hours. It took two aides holding each arm to assist Kathy in walking to the visiting area. The Zyprexa shut down the dopamine and her along with it. Kathy also was not very responsive to our presence and I doubt that she knew who we were. This is certainly not the way she entered the hospital when she was fully mobile and interactive.

Well, I guess this is one way to solve the problem. She wouldn't or couldn't bother anyone in this state! It was 2 weeks before they were ready to discharge her. The MCF agreed that she was ok to return in this condition.

When they released her, I had to have help getting her into the car. When she went in 2 weeks earlier, she was fully mobile, interactive, and played lovely piano chords. She has not played piano since. The medications had done further damage.

Her condition was absolutely not acceptable to me. I did not return Kathy to the MCF and I am disappointed that they even considered this condition acceptable.

Third Memory Care Facility

I had Kathy home long enough to start reducing the Zyprexa while we looked for another MCF. Slowly over time, she again became mobile and interactive, but sadly, she no longer played the piano. Fortunately, Zyprexa is not as difficult to discontinue as is Clonazapam.

We found a 5 resident MCF that was actually a 5 bedroom ranch house very close by. During the day, there were 2 aides, and 1 at night. I explained our previous bad experiences to the new doctor and my wish to minimize giving Kathy prescription drugs.

The medication of choice for this doctor was Depakote (Divalproex SOD 125mg Cap). I believe the initial prescription was for 2 capsules in the morning and 3 capsules in the evening. The doctor believed that Depakote would help with behavior and sleep issues. Later on it was actually increased from 5 to 7 capsules. However, at the 7 level, Kathy had ankle and foot swelling which had to be addressed. I didn't realize it, but Kathy was actually being given Depakote at the second MCF also.

Insomnia was a major problem here as well. She would sometimes go a couple days without sleeping. The doctor claimed that the Depakote aided sleep. However, it would have been very easy to plot a curve of insomnia versus Depakote. Insomnia increased with increasing Depakote. Maybe this is just a condition for Kathy. It is possible that the Clonazapam so damaged the GABA receptors that any medication that increases GABA quickly shuts down serotonin which is the precursor to the sleep regulating hormone melatonin. To this day, I can not give Kathy anything that increases GABA. That includes Lemon Balm, Passion Fruit, Taurine, Valerian, L-Theanine, etc. If I do, she will not sleep.

I would often pack a lunch and take Kathy to a nice park nearby. However, the last time I did that was a near disaster. I always knew when it was time to abort the mission and head back to the facility. Kathy would get a stern look on her face and typically say "Why did you do that", as if I was doing something wrong. At this point, I knew the clock was ticking and I needed to get back as fast as possible.

Too Late! When I tried to get her in the car, she started screaming and yelling like I was trying to rape her. People in another car in the parking lot were wondering what was going on. A lady came over and tried to help. As it turns out, she was a worker at another Assisted Living Facility. All was to no avail. Kathy proceeded to race across the parking lot and tried to climb a fence. When that didn't work, she headed down the sidewalk waving at cars and trying to stop them. I was scared to death that she would run out in front of one.

Fortunately, the direction she headed was toward the Fire Station. I was able to steer her to the station where I saw 3 firemen. They came to help and I told them about the situation. They restrained her (with difficulty) while I went back to get the car. It was not easy, but we were able to get her back into the car. By the time Kathy and I got back to the facility, she was happy and singing. Go figure!

Smallness again became an issue. Kathy is very active and the ranch house was just too constraining. She would try to move furniture, lamps, and pictures. Redirecting her became a common occurrence and Kathy became more agitated and combative. As a result, the Dapakote was increased and a second medication, Haldol, was added. Some details for this drug are:

*"**Haldol (Haloperidol)** is an antipsychotic. It blocks the effects of dopamine and increases its turnover rate, but may increase the risk of death when used to treat mental problems caused by dementia in elderly patients. Most of the deaths were linked to heart problems or infection. Haldol is not approved to treat mental problems caused by dementia."*

The combination of Haldol and Depakote was enough to shut Kathy down to the point where she could not even sit up by herself, let alone walk, and she was unresponsive to me. It was awful to see her just try to move one foot in front of the other. The situation continued to deteriorate as the medications continued to build up in her system. The doctor saw her but made no changes to the medication dosages.

That was it! I simply could not stand to see her in such an awful condition. I took her home and I never looked back. I finished off a bottle of wine that night because I knew that it was all on me now.

Back At Home

With some difficulty, I was able to get her home and in a chair in front of the TV. This is where she stayed unless I moved her. The first thing that happened is she voided on the chair. Then she wet the bed at night for the first several nights. When I took her to the bathroom to urinate, the urine was brownish and awful smelling. No wonder that they recommend liver and kidney tests every few months. The medications were such a toxic load.

Gradually, she was able to walk with assistance, and then by herself but had a couple of falls. It was odd at first. Kathy would walk around with her head back, looking upward. As a result, she would often run into furniture. This persisted for several weeks and I wondered if she would walk normally again.

The biggest concern of course was how I would get Kathy off the prescription drugs without significant bipolar behavior problems. To assist in doing this, I put 2 drops of Lavender essential oil on each wrist

4 times a day. I also wanted to charge her system with serotonin (the happy neurotransmitter). I did this by using L-Tryptophan, B6, and Nicotinic Acid mixed in applesauce about an hour before a meal, 4 times a day. L-Tryptophan has better absorption in the presence of carbohydrates with no protein. L-Tryptophan is the only amino acid that has a pathway to serotonin, and ultimately the sleep regulating hormone melatonin. If serotonin is shut down with GABA enhancing medication, insomnia can result. Normally the body uses L-Tryptophan to create niacin before being used to create serotonin. This is the reason that Nicotinic Acid is also added to the L-Tryptophan mixture. My understanding is that the form of niacin needed is Nicotinic Acid and not Niacinamide. The body does not recognize Niacinamide as a measure of adequate Niacin stores. I considered using 5-HTP instead of L-Tryptophan since it is further along the path to the creation of serotonin. However, I was concerned with the fact the body can not regulate the amount of 5-HTP as it does with L-Tryptophan. Thus, overdosing is possible, and is a major risk for anyone using SSRI's.

The transition off prescription drugs worked good enough so that we had no major behavioral problems. Fortunately, the medications that she was taking were not as addictive as Clonazapam, but withdrawal could still be a problem. Kathy was irritable and agitated at times, but not aggressive. To provide some relief, I had aides coming into our home 4 days a week for 4 hours per day. I later increases the aide times from 4 to 6 hours per day. Fortunately, Kathy's behavior was manageable and the the aides were able to take care of her without incident.

One of the most significant improvements in Kathy's behavior and sleep was the addition of hemp-derived CBD oil. At this writing, this was a legal supplement available at a local Health Food Store and online. Whereas cannabis has both THC oil (psychedelic action) and CBD oil, hemp essentially has only CBD oil. However, the CBD oil is the most effective for anxiety and many other ailments. These oils are cannabinoids and there are receptors for these throughout the body.

 If there was a circle with quadrants marked off for various moods, the effect of the CBD oil is to more the dot toward the good mood.

I give Kathy 10mg of CBD oil 4 times a day. Usually given at these times:

1. 7:00AM, Crushed banana, hemp oil, CBD oil, and partial capsules of curcumin and multivitamin/minerals.
2. 11:00AM, organic applesauce, and same as above.
3. 3:00PM, organic applesauce, and same as above.
4. 7:00PM, ground almond butter, raw honey, curcumin, and CBD oil.

The 10mg dosage just happened to be the amount in the capsules that I bought. At this dosage, 4 times a day seemed to work ok. It is unlikely that this is the optimum dosage. But, it is good enough for now.

Although Kathy now typically sleeps an uninterrupted 6 to 8 hours, there has been a downside. Because she is sleeping more soundly, sometimes she has urinary accidents, and some of those times wetting the bed. Usually, when she would only sleep 3 or 4 hours, I could usually catch her and take her to the bathroom. However, I am delighted that she sleeps longer, and hopefully the nighttime incontinence will stop.

During the day, urinary incontinence is rarely a problem. Kathy is toileted about every 3 hours. That has worked out very well. More often than not, Kathy will have a bowel movement along with the urination. However, this is not always and is the hardest to predict. Accidents do occasionally happen. It is for these instances that a hot-water vacuum cleaner comes in handy.

Kathy's current status is:
1. Home and off prescription drugs for 18 months.
2. Not aggressive and has minor irritation typically only when trying to get her in and out of the shower.
3. Sleep is essentially normal, but she has some issues with sleep apnea.
4. When in a deep sleep, sometimes has incontinence.
5. Takes 10mg CBD oil 4 times a day.
6. Takes curcumin, multivitamin, and coconut, hemp, and high DHA fish oils.
7. Must be toileted about every 3 hrs during the day, and at night if possible. I don't see any indication that she can be potty trained.
8. Fully mobile and we go for walks when weather permits.
9. Interactive and knows who I am.
10. Sometimes has a sadness mood that I haven't found a solution to yet.

Kathy seems to be getting better neuron by neuron. I read somewhere that it can take 10 years to recover from benzodiazopines. Kathy has too much damage to fully recover, but hopefully, at some point we can go out and do things together again.

Bottom Line

I believe Kathy has a chance for partial recovery because her Dementia root causes of Prescription Drugs and Gluten/Dairy have been addressed and eliminated. Without addressing and correcting the root causes, I doubt that recovery is possible with supplements alone.

It is helpful in the process of determining possible causes to have:

1.**Food Intolerance Test.** We chose the Mediator Release Test (MRT), which measures the mediator release of blood cells when exposed to various foods and food chemicals. **Reactive foods** are determined and can therefore be avoided to reduce **inflammation** in the body.

2. **Full Panel Blood Test and Hair Analysis.** We had to go to a Chiropractor to get this done. Family Doctor blood tests are typically very limited. This test should be completed to insure that there are no nutritional deficiencies that may affect brain

function, and the hair analysis can identify the presence of any elevated heavy metals.

3. **Genetic Analysis.** Sites like www.23andme.com may be helpful in determining if genetics is the underlying cause. Kathy has not had this test.

Finally, I continually try to avoid being blindsided by other potential problems. I avoid the "Dirty Dozen" vegetables and fruits that are laden with toxic chemicals and only eat those if organic. Although difficult, I also try to avoid GMO's.

After the root cause of the Dementia has been determined, it will likely require a major **Lifestyle Change**. Such a change is very difficult and can only be accomplished if those involved are "deadly serious".

Hoping for your success,
Richard

References:

1. Prescription Drug descriptions were obtained from www.Drugs.com and www.rxlist.com.
2. Danger of long-term use of Clonazapam was obtained from www.clonazapamaddictionhelp.com.
3. Brain damage effects were obtained from www.neuroskills.com.

Appendix
Prescription Drug Uses and Side Effects

Lisinopril (20mg)

Lisinopril is an ACE (angiotensin converting enzyme) inhibitor.

It is used to treat high blood pressure (hypertension) and is also used to treat congestive heart failure, or to improve survival after a heart attack.

Blood pressure (BP) will need to be checked often, and frequent blood tests may be needed.

Drinking alcohol can further lower your blood pressure and may increase certain side effects.

Avoid getting up too fast from a sitting or lying position, or dizziness may occur.

Severe Side effects:

Get emergency medical help if you have signs of an allergic reaction to lisinopril: hives; severe stomach pain, difficult breathing; swelling of your face, lips, tongue, or throat.

Call your doctor at once if you have: a light-headed feeling, like you might pass out, little or no urinating, fever, sore throat, high potassium - nausea, slow or unusual heart rate, weakness, loss of movement, kidney problems - little or no urinating, painful or difficult urination, swelling in your feet or ankles, feeling tired or short of breath, liver problems - nausea, upper stomach pain, itching, tired feeling, loss of appetite, dark urine, clay-colored stools, jaundice (yellowing of the skin or eyes).

Common Side Effects:
Headache, dizziness, cough, chest pain.

This is not a complete list of side effects and others may occur.

Hydrochorothiazide (12.5mg)

HCTZ (hydrochlorothiazide) is a thiazide diuretic (water pill) that helps prevent your body from absorbing too much salt, which can cause fluid retention. It treats fluid retention (edema) in people with congestive heart failure, cirrhosis of the liver, or kidney disorders, or edema.

Major Side Effects:

Abdominal or stomach pain, back, leg, or stomach pains, black, tarry stools, bleeding gums, blistering, peeling, or loosening of the skin, bloating, blood in the urine or stools, bloody urine, blue lips and fingernails, blurred vision, burning, crawling, itching, numbness, prickling, "pins and needles", or tingling feelings, chest pain, chills, clay-colored stools, cloudy urine, cold sweats, confusion, constipation, cough or hoarseness, coughing that sometimes produces a pink frothy sputum, coughing up blood, plus 70 more Side Effects

Minor Side Effects:

Cramping, decreased interest in sexual intercourse, difficulty having a bowel movement (stool), feeling of constant movement of self or surroundings, hair loss or thinning of the hair, inability to have or keep an erection, increased sensitivity of the skin to sunlight, loss in sexual ability, desire, drive, or performance, muscle spasm, pinpoint red or purple spots on the skin, redness or other discoloration of the skin, restlessness, sensation of spinning, severe sunburn, weakness.

Clonazapam (Klonopin) (0.5mg)

Clonazepam is a benzodiazepine. It affects chemicals in the brain that may be unbalanced.The precise mechanism by which clonazepam exerts its antiseizure and antipanic effects is unknown, although it is believed to be related to its ability to enhance the activity of gamma aminobutyric acid (GABA), the major inhibitory neurotransmitter in the central nervous system.

It is also used to treat panic disorder (including agoraphobia)

Clonazepam may be habit-forming. Misuse of habit-forming medicine can cause addiction, overdose, or death.

Clonazepam should be used for only a short time. Do not take this medication for longer than 9 weeks without your doctor's advice. Use of this medicine long-term may require frequent medical tests.

Memory loss is a common side effect of clonazepam use.

Do not stop using clonazepam suddenly. Unpleasant withdrawal symptoms, including a seizure (convulsions) could result. Ask your doctor how to safely stop using this medicine.

More Common Side Effects:

Body aches or pain, chills, cough, difficulty breathing, discouragement, dizziness, ear congestion, feeling sad or empty, fever, headache, irritability, lack of appetite, loss of interest or pleasure, loss of voice, nasal congestion, poor coordination, runny nose, shakiness and unsteady walk, sleepiness or unusual drowsiness, sneezing, sore throat, tiredness, trouble concentrating, trouble sleeping, unsteadiness, trembling, or other problems with muscle control or coordination, unusual tiredness or weakness.

Less Common Side Effects:

Being forgetful, bladder pain, bloody or cloudy urine, change in speech, diarrhea, difficult, burning, or painful urination, frequent urge to urinate, general feeling of discomfort or illness, joint pain, loss of appetite, lower back or side pain, mood or mental changes, muscle aches and pains, nausea, nervousness, problems in urination or increase in the amount of urine, shivering, slurred speech, sore throat, sweating, trouble speaking.

Pyridostigmine (Mestinon) BR 60mg Tablet

Mestinon is an orally active cholinesterase inhibitor. Pyridostigmine bromide inhibits the destruction of acetylcholine by cholinesterase and thereby permits freer transmission of nerve impulses across the neuromuscular junction. **Severe Side Effects:** Severe allergic reactions (rash; hives; itching; difficulty breathing; tightness in the chest; swelling of the mouth, face, lips, or tongue); diarrhea; fainting; increased production of saliva; increased sweating; muscle weakness; nausea; small pupils; stomach cramps; trouble breathing; vision changes; vomiting; weakness. This is not a complete list of all side effects that may occur.

Divalproex SOD(Depakote) 125mg Cap (DB)

Divalproex sodium affects chemicals in the body that may be involved in causing seizures. It is also used to treat manic episodes related to bipolar disorder (manic depression), and to prevent migraine headaches. Unfortunately, the anticonvulsant medication has been linked to suicide, liver toxicity, and pancreatitis. Divalproex works by increasing the amount of the neurotransmitter gamma amminobutyric acid (GABA) in the brain.   .

Major Side Effects. More common:

Black, tarry stools, bleeding gums, bloating or swelling of the face, arms, hands, lower legs, or feet, blood in the urine or stools, confusion, cough or hoarseness, crying, delusions, dementia' depersonalization, diarrhea, difficult or labored breathing, dysphoria, euphoria, fever or chills, general feeling of discomfort or illness, headache, joint pain, loss of appetite, lower back or side pain, mental depression, muscle aches and pains, nausea, nervousness, painful or difficult urination, paranoia, pinpoint red spots on the skin, quick to react or overreact emotionally, rapid weight gain, rapidly changing moods, runny nose, shakiness in the legs, arms, hands, or feet, shivering, sleepiness or unusual drowsiness, sore throat, sweating, tightness in the chest, tingling of the hands or feet, trembling or shaking of the hands or feet, trouble sleeping, unusual bleeding or bruising, unusual tiredness or weakness, unusual weight gain or loss, vomiting

Less common:

Abnormal dreams, absence of or decrease in body movement, anxiety, bloody nose, blurred vision, bruising burning, crawling, itching, numbness, prickling, "pins and needles", or tingling feelings, change in personality, change in walking and balance, changes in patterns and rhythms of speech, chest pain, chills, cloudy urine, clumsiness or unsteadiness, cold sweats, constipation, darkened urine, degenerative disease of the joint, difficulty with moving, dizziness, dizziness, faintness, or lightheadedness when getting up from a lying or sitting position suddenly, dry mouth, excessive muscle tone, fast, irregular, pounding, or racing heartbeat or pulse, feeling of warmth or heat, flushing or redness of the skin, especially on the face and neck, frequent urge to urinate, heavy non-menstrual vaginal bleeding, hyperventilation, increased need to urinate, indigestion, lack of coordination, **large, flat, blue or purplish patches in the skin,** leg cramps, lip smacking or puckering, **loss of bladder control,** loss of strength or energy, multiple swollen and inflamed skin lesions, muscle pain or stiffness, muscle tension or tightness, normal menstrual bleeding occurring earlier, possibly lasting longer than expected, pains in the stomach, side, or abdomen, possibly radiating to the back, passing urine more often, pounding in the ears, puffing of the cheeks, rapid or worm-like movements of the tongue, rapid weight gain, restlessness, seeing, hearing, or feeling things that are not there, shakiness and unsteady walk, slurred speech, small red or purple spots on the skin, sweating, swollen joints, trouble with speaking, twitching, uncontrolled chewing movements, uncontrolled movements of the arms and legs, unsteadiness, trembling, or other problems with muscle control or coordination, vomiting of blood or material that looks like coffee grounds, yellow eyes or skin

Minor Side Effects were also observed but are not presented here.

Venlafaxine HCL (Effexor) 37.5 mg Tablet

Venlafaxine is an antidepressant in a group of drugs called selective serotonin and norepinephrine reuptake inhibitors (SSNRIs). Venlafaxine affects chemicals in the brain that may be unbalanced in people with depression. It is used to treat major depressive disorder, anxiety, and panic disorder.

Major Side Effects
More common:
High blood pressure, lack or loss of strength, severe headache, sweating
Less common:
Blurred vision, chest pain, fast or irregular heartbeat, mood or mental changes, ringing or buzzing in the ears, suicidal thoughts
Rare:
Actions that are out of control, convulsions, high fever, high or low blood pressure, irritability, itching or skin rash, lightheadedness or fainting, especially when getting up suddenly from a sitting or lying position, menstrual changes, nervousness, problems with urinating or holding urine, severe muscle stiffness, talking, feeling, and acting with

excitement that you cannot control, trouble breathing, unusually pale skin

Incidence not known:

Agitation, bloody, black, or tarry stools, bloody stool or urine, confusion, dark urine, decreased frequency or amount of urine, diarrhea, drowsiness, fever, general feeling of tiredness or weakness, headache, increased thirst, light-colored stools, muscle cramps, spasms, or pain, nausea or vomiting, nosebleeds, overactive reflexes, poor coordination, red or purple spots on skin, restlessness, shivering, stomach pain on upper right side, swelling of the face, lower legs, ankles, hands, or fingers, trembling or shaking that is hard to control, twitching, unusual bruising, unusual tiredness or weakness, vomiting of blood or material that looks like coffee grounds, yellow eyes or skin

Minor Side Effects were observed but are not included here.

Amantadine 50mg/5 ml Syrup

Amantadine prevents and treats certain types of flu. It is used to treat Parkinson disease and uncontrolled muscle movements caused by some medicines. How amantadine works against Parkinson disease is not known.

Common Side Effects:

Appetite loss; blurred vision; constipation; diarrhea; dizziness; drowsiness; dry mouth or nose; headache; lightheadedness; nausea; strange dreams; tiredness; trouble sleeping.

Severe Side Effects:

Severe allergic reactions (rash; hives; itching; difficulty breathing; tightness in the chest; swelling of the mouth, face, lips, or tongue); aggression; agitation; confusion; depression; fainting; fast or irregular heartbeat; fever; hallucinations; memory loss; mental or mood changes; muscle problems (eg, spasms, uncontrolled movements); paranoid thoughts; personality changes; seizures; severe or persistent drowsiness or trouble sleeping; shortness of breath; sore throat; swelling of hands, legs, feet, or ankles; thoughts of suicide; trouble urinating; unusual anxiety or irritability; vision changes. This is not a complete list of all side effects that may occur.

Haldol (Haloperidol) 1/2 of 2mg Tablet

Haldol is an antipsychotic. It blocks the effects of dopamine and increases its turnover rate, but may increase the risk of death when used to treat mental problems caused by dementia in elderly patients. Most of the deaths were linked to heart problems or infection. Haldol is not approved to treat mental problems caused by dementia.

Common Side Effects:

Constipation; diarrhea; dizziness; drowsiness; dry mouth; headache; loss of appetite; nausea; restlessness; stomach upset; trouble sleeping.

Severe Side Effects:

Severe allergic reactions (rash; hives; itching; difficulty breathing; tightness in the chest; swelling of the mouth, face, lips, or tongue); blurred vision or other vision changes; chest pain; confusion; dark urine; decreased or difficult urination; decreased sexual ability; dehydration; difficulty speaking or swallowing; drooling; enlarged breasts; excessive or unusual sweating; fainting; fast or irregular heartbeat; fever, chills, or persistent sore throat; hallucinations; mental or mood changes (eg, abnormal thinking, agitation, anxiety, depression); missed menstrual period or other menstrual changes; nipple discharge; prolonged, painful erection; rigid or stiff muscles; seizures; severe or persistent dizziness, headache, or vomiting; shortness of breath or unusual cough; shuffling walk; uncontrolled muscle movements (eg, of the arms, legs, tongue, jaw, cheeks; tremors; twitching); yellowing of the skin or eyes.

Common Side Effects:

Appetite loss; blurred vision; constipation; diarrhea; dizziness; drowsiness; dry mouth or nose; headache; lightheadedness; nausea; strange dreams; tiredness; trouble sleeping.

Severe Side Effects:

Severe allergic reactions (rash; hives; itching; difficulty breathing; tightness in the chest; swelling of the mouth, face, lips, or tongue); aggression; agitation; confusion; depression; fainting; fast or irregular heartbeat; fever; hallucinations; memory loss; mental or mood changes; muscle problems (eg, spasms, uncontrolled movements); paranoid thoughts; personality changes; seizures; severe or persistent drowsiness or trouble sleeping; shortness of breath; sore throat; swelling of hands, legs, feet, or ankles; thoughts of suicide; trouble urinating; unusual anxiety or irritability; vision changes. This is not a complete list of all side effects that may occur.

Haldol (Haloperidol) 1/2 of 2mg Tablet

Haldol is an antipsychotic. It blocks the effects of dopamine and increases its turnover rate, but may increase the risk of death when used to treat mental problems caused by dementia in elderly patients. Most of the deaths were linked to heart problems or infection. Haldol is not approved to treat mental problems caused by dementia.

Common Side Effects:

Constipation; diarrhea; dizziness; drowsiness; dry mouth; headache; loss of appetite; nausea; restlessness; stomach upset; trouble sleeping.

Severe Side Effects:

Severe allergic reactions (rash; hives; itching; difficulty breathing; tightness in the chest; swelling of the mouth, face, lips, or tongue); blurred vision or other vision changes; chest pain; confusion; dark urine; decreased or difficult urination; decreased sexual ability; dehydration; difficulty speaking or swallowing; drooling; enlarged breasts; excessive or unusual sweating; fainting; fast or irregular heartbeat; fever, chills, or persistent sore throat; hallucinations; mental or mood changes (eg, abnormal thinking, agitation, anxiety, depression); missed menstrual period or other menstrual changes; nipple discharge; prolonged, painful erection; rigid or stiff muscles; seizures; severe or persistent dizziness, headache, or vomiting; shortness of breath or unusual cough; shuffling walk; uncontrolled muscle movements (eg, of the arms, legs, tongue, jaw, cheeks; tremors; twitching); yellowing of the skin or eyes.

This is not a complete list of all side effects that may occur.